THE 2023 ELIMINATION DIET COOKBOOK

Simple And Quick Elimination Diet Recipes For An Optimal State Of Health

By

Dr. Sophia Perry

Copyright@2022 by Dr. Sophia Perry

TABLE OF CONTENTS

CHAPTER 1

FOOD INTOLERANCES, FOOD ALLERGIES, CELIAC DISEASE, AND FOOD INSENSITIVITY

Chances are that you or someone you know has experienced unpleasant symptoms after a meal or snack. Perhaps you had sneezing, wheezing, rashes, brain fog, joint pain, nausea, bloating, diarrhea, or another symptom. This may have led you to believe you have a food allergy, which you may have. However, you could have a food intolerance, celiac disease, or a food sensitivity. This is significant because some of the reactions can range from simply irritating to life-threatening.

FOOD INTOLERANCES

Food intolerance is the inability to process or digest certain foods. The most common food reaction appears to be lactose intolerance. Our ability to digest dairy diminishes as we age. This is because as we get older, our intestines produce less of the enzyme (lactase) that breaks down lactose, a type of sugar found in milk and dairy products. As a result, there is more lactose in the digestive tract, which can cause stomach bloating, inflammation, and diarrhea. According to studies, only about 35% of people worldwide can digest lactose after the age of seven or eight. Lactose intolerance is not a serious disease, but it can be very uncomfortable.

FOOD ALLERGIES

When someone has a true allergic reaction, the body's immune system overreacts to a seemingly harmless substance — in this case, a food. The classic example is potentially fatal difficulty breathing and low blood pressure after exposure to peanuts or seafood. Food allergies can strike at any age, including middle age.

If you suspect you have a food allergy, consider allergy testing and treatment, especially if your symptoms are severe (significant rashes, feeling of passing out, facial swelling, and problems breathing). It is prudent to read ingredient labels carefully. And having epinephrine shots on hand in case of accidental ingestion or contact with the food in question is critical and can save lives.

CELIAC DISEASE

Celiac disease affects about 1% of the Western population. In this autoimmune condition, the ingestion of gluten initiates a complex inflammatory reaction that can make people with celiac disease very sick. Celiac disease is not a true allergy; eating gluten once does not cause an immediate life-threatening problem. However, prolonged and continuous ingestion can cause diarrhea, weight loss, and malnutrition.

Avoiding gluten is the only solution to this problem. Gluten can be found in grains such as wheat, rye, barley, semolina, bulgur, and farina. Gluten is also found in many processed foods. People with celiac disease must also be careful about cross-contamination, when a gluten-free food comes into contact with a gluten-containing food.

FOOD SENSITIVITIES

After eating certain foods, a large part of the population experiences symptoms that are not related to food intolerances, food allergies, or celiac disease. These are referred to as food sensitivities. Though there is some debate about what happens in the body of someone who has a food sensitivity, it appears that exposure to specific foods may cause an immune reaction that causes a variety of symptoms. The symptoms, which include joint pain, stomach pain, fatigue, rashes, and brain fog, are not life threatening, but they can be quite disruptive. Gluten is probably the most well-known allergen.

A process of careful observation and experimentation is the most effective tool we have for identifying food sensitivities. The current gold standard for determining what may be causing symptoms is to remove certain foods suspected of causing reactions from the diet for two to four weeks, reintroduce them one by one, and monitor for symptoms.

CHAPTER 2

THE ELIMINATION DIET

HOW TO DO AN ELIMINATION DIET AND WHY

Elimination diets are the gold standard for dietary testing to identify food intolerances, sensitivities, and allergies. They eliminate certain foods that are known to cause unpleasant symptoms and reintroduce them later while testing for symptoms.

Elimination diets have been used by allergists and registered dietitians for decades to help people eliminate foods that are not well tolerated.

WHAT IS AN ELIMINATION DIET?

An elimination diet involves removing foods from your diet that you suspect your body can't tolerate well. The foods are then gradually reintroduced while you keep an eye out for any reactions.

It is used to identify which foods are causing symptoms in people with celiac disease, a sensitive gut, food allergies, or food intolerance. In this way, bloating, gas, diarrhea, constipation, and nausea symptoms may be reduced by an elimination diet.There are various elimination diets that all involve eating or avoiding particular food groups. However, if you have a known or suspected food allergy, then you should only try an elimination diet under the supervision of a medical professional. Reintroducing a food allergen may trigger a dangerous condition called anaphylaxis.If you suspect you have a food allergy, check with your doctor before starting an elimination diet. Symptoms of an allergy include rashes, hives, swelling and difficulty breathing.

HOW DOES IT WORK?

An elimination diet is divided into two phases: elimination and reintroduction.

THE ELIMINATION PHASE

In the elimination phase, foods are eliminated for a brief period of time usually 2-3 weeks from which you believe your symptoms may be caused. Eliminate foods that you believe your body can't handle as well as those known for bringing on unpleasant symptoms.

Among these foods are nuts, dairy, citrus fruits, nightshade vegetables, corn, soy, wheat, foods containing gluten, pork, eggs, and seafood.

This phase allows you to ascertain whether your symptoms are brought on by certain foods or something else. It is best to call your doctor if your symptoms persist after cutting out certain foods for two to three weeks.

THE REINTRODUCTION PHASE

The next phase is the reintroduction phase, in which you slowly bring eliminated foods back into your diet.

Each food group should be introduced individually, over 2–3 days, while looking for symptoms. Some symptoms to watch for include:

1. Rashes and skin changes

2. Joint pain

3. Headaches or migraines

4. Fatigue

5. Difficulty sleeping

6. Changes in breathing

7. Bloating

8. Stomach pain or cramps

9. Changes in bowel habits

If you have no symptoms while reintroducing a food group, you can assume that it is safe to eat and move on to the next food group.

However, if you experience negative symptoms like those listed above, you have identified a trigger food and should eliminate it from your diet.

The entire process, including elimination, takes about 5-6 weeks.

HOW DOES AN ELIMINATION DIET WORK?

The first step for me is to include the patient in the process. It is not simple to exclude meals and then challenge them, so dedication to the process is essential.

1. KEEP A TWO-WEEK FOOD JOURNAL.

When I say "detailed," I mean it. You wouldn't type "salad" for lunch. Instead, put "baby spinach, cherry tomatoes, red pepper, feta cheese, chicken breast, olive oil and vinegar." Begin by reading labels and adding anything notable. On top of wheat, did the crackers you just ate include eggs, dairy, and soy? Were there garlic or onion flavorings in the dishes that made you sick? I tell my patients that they must assist me by acting as detectives in their own kitchens and freezers.

I also ask my participants to keep a journal of how they feel a few hours after eating, noting any symptoms such as bloating, intestinal pain, rashes, or hives. These might be useful indicators when determining which meals to avoid and which to challenge later on.

The food diary is especially important since individuals don't always pay attention to what they eat. For example, they may tell me that they don't consume a lot of dairy products, implying that dairy isn't likely to be causing their symptoms. However, their meal journal reveals that they eat yogurt for breakfast, cheese for lunch, and ice cream for dessert. Milk may also be found in unexpected places such as baked products, crackers, and confectionery.

2. EXAMINE THE FOOD DIARY FOR TRENDS.

For example:

- Wheat
- Dairy
- Eggs
- Soy
- Peanuts
- Nutty trees (e.g. walnuts, almonds, cashews)
- Shellfish (e.g. crab, shrimp, lobster) (e.g. crab, shrimp, lobster)
- Fish
- Sesame

When the food diary is finished, I ask two important questions:

a. What meals do you consume the most frequently?

b. Which of the following common food allergies feature regularly in your diet?

Next, I compare the diary to the findings of the food allergy test (IgE testing may be done concurrently with the food diary) to generate a list of items to avoid and challenge. We begin with the meals that are most likely to cause an issue and work our way down to the foods that are least likely to cause an issue.

3. SYSTEMATICALLY ELIMINATE POTENTIAL PROBLEM FOODS.

To begin, I recommend that patients eliminate one meal from their diet for eight days. I normally have my patients do this from Saturday to Saturday since it's simpler for them to begin on a day when they're not working.

Substitutions

In certain circumstances, patients find that acceptable substitutes or meals that imitate a texture or flavor are beneficial. I suggest the following:

- Dairy milk alternatives: Coconut milk, almond milk, oat milk, flax milk, rice milk, hemp milk or other mammalian milk if tolerated (goat, sheep, even camel milk).

- Dairy cheese alternatives: Avocado, dairy-free cheese substitutes, feta (made from sheep's milk, if tolerated).

- Wheat bread alternatives: Gluten-free bread made from rice, sorghum, amaranth, quinoa and corn, corn tortillas.

- Egg alternatives: Flax egg (one tablespoon flaxseed combined with three tablespoons water), tofu (if not eliminating soy).

- Peanut alternatives: Tree nuts including almonds, cashews, walnuts, pecans and peanut butter alternatives like soy-based butter, legume-based butter, seed butter.

- Tree nut alternatives: Peanuts, soy-based butter, legume-based butter, seed butter.
- Fish alternatives: Poultry, red meats, vegan fish-sauce substitutes (for cooking).
- Shellfish alternatives: Crab alternatives (made with whitefish and wheat).
- Soy sauce alternatives: Coconut aminos.
- Soybeans: Chickpeas.

Identifying the culprit(s) If you feel better and your symptoms begin to improve after eliminating a certain meal for eight days, it's a strong indication that what you've removed is causing your issue. Some individuals, however, do not detect a difference when they remove the item; they only see a genuine improvement in their symptoms when they reintroduce the suspect food during the challenge stage.

4. REINTRODUCE POTENTIALLY PROBLEMATIC FOODS GRADUALLY.

Following the elimination phase, I urge my patients to reintroduce a previously excluded meal via a method called as a challenge. They do this challenge over the course of a weekend in case the reintroduction effects are unpleasant and interfere with work.

To reintroduce the removed meal, a patient will consume it twice in one day, generally in quick succession. So, if you're testing milk, drink a glass of milk first thing in the morning and then wait an hour. If you have symptoms, we will stop there. Milk is now one of your problem meals. Depending on the scenario, we may still remove and challenge a few more items.

If you have no symptoms after the first glass of milk, I would recommend that you consume another glass. If you're still feeling well after many hours, we may conclude that milk isn't a problem meal and move on to the next one on the list.

ADVANTAGES OF THE ELIMINATION DIET

Elimination diets help you discover which foods cause uncomfortable symptoms so you can remove them from your diet. However, an elimination diet has many other benefits, including:

1. IT MAY HELP WITH IRRITABLE BOWEL SYNDROME (IBS).

Irritable bowel syndrome (IBS) is a prevalent digestive illness that affects 10-15% of the world's population.

An elimination diet helps many individuals with IBS symptoms such as bloating, stomach cramps, and gas. In one research, 150 participants with IBS were randomly assigned to either an elimination diet that omitted trigger foods or a phony elimination diet that excluded the same amount of items but not those associated with unpleasant symptoms.

People who adhered to the elimination diet decreased their symptoms by 10%, while those who adhered to the diet the best reduced their symptoms by up to 26%.

2. IT MAY BENEFIT THOSE SUFFERING FROM EOSINOPHILIC ESOPHAGITIS.

Eosinophilic esophagitis (EE) is a chronic illness in which allergens inflame the esophagus, the tube that transports food from the mouth to the stomach. People with EE have trouble swallowing dry, thick meals, which increases their risk of choking.

Elimination diets have been demonstrated in several trials to be useful in relieving EE symptoms. It has helped over 75% of 146 people with EE have considerably reduced symptoms and inflammation.

3. IT MAY ALLEVIATE ADHD SYMPTOMS.

Attention deficit hyperactivity disorder (ADHD) is a behavioral disease that affects 3-5% of all children and adults.

Elimination diets have been demonstrated in studies to help with ADHD symptoms. One study examined 20 research that limited certain meals in order to treat ADHD symptoms. Researchers discovered that exclusion diets reduced ADHD symptoms in children who were food sensitive.

However, except under the supervision of a medical expert, children should not follow an elimination diet.

Many vital nutrients that are needed for developing children are restricted on elimination diets, and long-term restriction may impede their development.

4. IT HAS THE POTENTIAL TO IMPROVE SKIN CONDITIONS SUCH AS ECZEMA.

Eczema is a skin disorder characterized by red, itchy, cracked, and irritated skin. Although there are several causes of eczema, many patients find that specific foods aggravate their symptoms.

Several studies have suggested that elimination diets may help to alleviate eczema symptoms. An exclusion diet lowered symptoms and helped identify trigger items in one trial of 15 eczema patients.

5. IT MAY HELP WITH CHRONIC MIGRAINES.

Chronic migraines affect over 2-3 million individuals in the United States alone. Although the origins of migraines are unknown, research have suggested that inflammation may be a trigger.

An elimination diet, which eliminates inflammatory foods, has been demonstrated to alleviate persistent migraines.

In one research, 28 women and 2 men who had regular migraines followed an exclusion diet for six weeks, which reduced the frequency of headache episodes from nine to six.

CHAPTER 3

RECOMMENDATIONS AND RECIPES

You don't have to sacrifice flavor or satisfaction on an elimination diet. Below are our recommendations for foods to enjoy on an elimination diet, as well as which foods to avoid.

VEGETABLE:

Enjoy: Low-sugar foods include berries, green apples, lemons and limes.

Avoid: High-sugar foods like bananas, grapes, pineapple, mango or dried fruits.

BEEF & CHICKEN:

Enjoy: Organic, pasture-raised poultry and meat; pasture-raised eggs.

Avoid: Conventionally farmed animal proteins combined with any processed meats.

FISH & SEAFOOD:

Enjoy: Wild-caught fish; sustainably harvested shellfish.

Avoid: All farm-raised seafood and bigger fish including tuna and swordfish.

FATS & OILS:

Enjoy: A range of excellent quality oils, including cold-pressed olive oil, avocado oil, coconut oil, grass-fed ghee and lard; additional sources of healthy fat include olives, coconut goods, avocado and tahini.

Avoid: All trans fats and processed seed and vegetable oils including canola, sunflower, soybean and corn oil.

NUTS & SEEDS:

Enjoy: A variety of nuts and seeds.
Avoid: Peanuts.

DAIRY & DAIRY ALTERNATIVES:

Enjoy: Grass-fed butter and ghee; unsweetened dairy substitutes such as nut and seed milks.

Avoid: All other dairy-containing foods.

BEANS & LEGUMES:

If vegetarian or vegan, enjoy (in restricted amounts): Legumes such as black beans, chickpeas, lentils or kidney beans.

Avoid: All non-organic soy products and all processed soy products including soy milk, soybean oil and tofu.

GLUTEN & GRAINS:

Enjoy: Grain-free choices include meals prepared with almond flour and coconut flour.

Avoid: All gluten, grains and gluten-free meals, including rice, quinoa or oats.

SUGAR & SWEETENER:

Enjoy: Small quantities of pure monk fruit (no erythritol) and pure stevia (no erythritol or natural flavors) (no erythritol or natural flavors).

Avoid: All additional forms of sugar.

BEVERAGES:

Enjoy: Plenty of filtered water, herbal tea, seltzer, sparkling water and bone broth; cold-pressed, vegetable-only juices; up to one cup per day of organic coffee, matcha or green tea.

Avoid: All sweetened beverages including juices, energy drinks, sweet tea & soda; drinks with artificial sweeteners; alcohol.

RECIPES

ALMOND COCOA SMOOTHIE

2 servings

2 cups unsweetened almond milk

1 scoop vegan protein powder

1 small avocado

1 tbsp cocoa powder

1 teaspoon almond extract

½ cup ice cubes

Stevia, to taste (optional)

1-2 cups chopped kale, packed loosely

Rice, peas, and hemp are examples of common varieties. Should be sweetened with stevia or left unsweetened entirely. 1 scoop should contain 17g protein.

Directions

1. Place all of the ingredients in a blender in the order listed.

2. In a blender, combine all ingredients and blend on low to high speed until smooth.

3. To achieve the desired thickness, add more or less ice.

ALMOND MILK

3 servings

½ cup raw almonds

4 cup purified water

2 tbsp pure maple syrup (optional)

a pinch of sea salt

Directions

1. Soak almonds and 1 cup purified water in a blender at room temperature for 6 hours.

2. Drain off the water and rinse the almonds thoroughly under running water after they have soaked.

3. Return almonds to blender with 3 cups purified water, maple syrup (optional), and sea salt. Blend on high for 2-3 minutes.

4. Squeeze out any remaining liquid with a cheesecloth or strainer with fine holes.

Tips: The leftover almond pieces can be added to oatmeal, muffins, or anything else you can think of to boost the fiber content.

APPLE CINNAMON AMARANTH PORRIDGE

4 servings

2 cups water

1 cup amaranth

1 large apple, skin on, cored and diced

¼ teaspoon ground cinnamon

½ teaspoon sea salt

Directions

1. Combine all of the ingredients in a medium saucepan and bring to a boil. Stir frequently.

2. Reduce heat to low and cover for 20-25 minutes, or until amaranth is soft.

Tips: This can be made the night before and reheated in the morning. Refrigerate leftovers in an airtight glass container for up to 5 days.

Serve with coconut or almond milk to taste. If more sweetness is desired, a small amount of stevia can be added. Serve with walnuts if desired.

BAKED CHICKEN WITH CABBAGE, CARROTS, AND ONIONS

4 servings

4 halved chicken breasts (bone-in, skin-on)

1 chopped head cabbage

1 large onion cut into eighths

1 pound baby carrot bag

1 tsp kosher salt (divided)

1 teaspoon ground black pepper

2-3 fresh rosemary sprigs, finely minced (2-3 teaspoons)

1 garlic head, cloves separated and unpeeled (or 4-5 teaspoons minced garlic)

¼ cup extra-virgin olive oil 1 lemon, quartered

3 tablespoons vinegar (red wine)

Directions

1. Heat the oven to 450° F.

2. Place the chicken, cabbage, onion, and carrots in a 12 x 16-inch glass dish or roasting pan. Mix ½ teaspoon salt, ½ teaspoon pepper, and ½ teaspoon rosemary in a small bowl. Sprinkle over the chicken and vegetables. Toss gently.

3. Arrange the chicken on top of the vegetables, skin side up. On top of the vegetables, sprinkle with garlic cloves and a quartered lemon.

4. In a separate small bowl, whisk together the oil, vinegar, and the remaining ½ teaspoon salt and pepper. Drizzle the sauce over the chicken and vegetables.

5. Bake for 50 minutes at 350°F. The chicken should be browned and thoroughly cooked. Vegetables should be soft.

Tips: Instead of using chicken breast halves, consider roasting a whole chicken.

BAKED SALMON WITH DILL

4 servings

4 fillets of salmon (5 ounces each)

4 teaspoons fresh dill, chopped

4 teaspoons extra virgin olive oil

¼ teaspoon salt

¼ teaspoon pepper

Directions

1. Heat the oven to 375° F.

2. Line or oil a cookie sheet with parchment paper. Pour in the salmon.

3. Combine olive oil, dill, salt, and pepper in a small bowl and brush over salmon.

4. Bake the salmon for 12-15 minutes at 350°F.

BALSAMIC ROASTED BEETS

2 servings

1 bunch trimmed beets (about 4 beets)

1 tbsp balsamic vinegar

2 pinches sea salt

2 pinches black pepper

Directions

1. Preheat the oven to 400° F.

2. Gently scrub beets and pat dry. Wrap in foil and bake until tender (about 1 hour). Let cool before peeling and dicing.

3. Toss beets with balsamic vinegar, sea salt, and pepper in a medium bowl, and serve.

Tips: Make more beets than you need and store them in the fridge for later in the week (salads, snacks, side dishes, etc.).

BROILED LAMB CHOPS WITH ROSEMARY

4 servings

4 lamb chops (lean)

2 teaspoon olive oil

1 teaspoon dried rosemary

1 tbsp fresh rosemary

½ teaspoon sea salt

½ teaspoon pepper

Directions

1. Preheat the broiler.

2. Drizzle oil over lamb chops and rub to coat.

3. Combine the salt, pepper, and dried rosemary in a small bowl and season both sides of the lamb chops. Rub spices into the chops.

4. Transfer the lamb to a broiler pan and broil for 8-10 minutes. During the cooking process, flip once. When done, the lamb should be slightly pink in the center.

CHIA SEED APPLESAUCE BREAD

16 servings

1 cup teff flour

1 pound rice flour

3 tablespoons chia seed

1 teaspoon. baking soda

½ teaspoon ground cinnamon

¼ teaspoon nutmeg

¼ teaspoon salt

1 cup applesauce, unsweetened

1 tablespoon melted coconut oil

1 pound brown rice syrup

3 teaspoon apple butter

1 teaspoon vanilla extract, pure

1 large peeled, cored, and chopped apple

Egg replacer:

13 cup of water

1 tbsp. ground flax seed

Directions

1. Make the egg replacer by combining ground flax and water. Allow 5 minutes for the mixture to gel.

2. Combine dry ingredients in a large mixing bowl (teff and rice flours, chia seed, baking soda, cinnamon, salt, and nutmeg). Wet ingredients should be combined in a smaller bowl (applesauce, melted coconut oil, brown rice syrup, apple butter and vanilla extract).

3. Mix the wet and dry ingredients together. Mix in the apple chunks.

4. Pour the mixture into an oiled 9-inch square baking pan. Bake for 30 minutes at 350° F.

5. When completely cool, cut into 16 servings.

Tips: Oat flour can be used in place of rice flour, and maple syrup, agave nectar, or fruit juice concentrate can be used in place of brown rice syrup.

CHOPPED SALAD WITH TUNA

4 servings

Salad:

1 can (12 ounce) tuna, drained and separated

1 cup chopped cucumber

1 cup tomato, chopped

1 avocado, chopped

1 cup celery, chopped

½ cup radishes, chopped

4 cups romaine lettuce, chopped

¼ cup extra virgin olive oil for dressing

¼ cup freshly squeezed lime juice

4 minced garlic cloves

1 teaspoon ground black pepper

1 teaspoon coarse sea salt

Directions

1. Combine tuna, cucumber, tomato, avocado, celery, radishes, and lettuce in a large mixing bowl.

2. Combine the dressing ingredients in a mixing bowl. Pour over the salad and gently toss to coat.

3. Serve right away.

CILANTRO LIME CAULIFLOWER RICE

6 servings

1 cauliflower head (24 ounces or 6 cups chopped)

1 tbsp olive oil (extra virgin)

2 garlic cloves

¼ teaspoon sea salt 2 diced scallions

¼ teaspoon black pepper

3 tbsp fresh lime juice (the juice of 12 limes)

¼ cup chopped fresh cilantro

Directions

1. Rinse and pat dry the cauliflower. In a food processor, chop into florets and grate. If you don't have a food processor, grate the cauliflower with a box grater. The

cauliflower should have the consistency of rice or couscous.

2. Heat the olive oil, garlic, and scallions in a large skillet over medium heat. Cook for 3-4 minutes.

3. Raise the heat to medium-high and add the cauliflower. Remove from heat and transfer to a large mixing bowl after 5-6 minutes (before cauliflower gets mushy).

2.Add sea salt, pepper, lime juice, and cilantro to taste.

COCONUT CHICKEN

4 servings

2 tbsp extra virgin olive oil or organic virgin coconut oil

½ cup chopped onion

2 cloves minced garlic

2 cup diced fresh tomatoes

1 pound boneless chicken breasts, cut into strips

1 tbsp curry powder

⅓ cup coconut milk

⅓ cup water

⅛ teaspoon ground cinnamon

5 fresh basil leaves, chopped for garnish

½ teaspoon salt

¼ teaspoon freshly ground pepper

Directions

1. In a large skillet, heat the oil over medium heat. Cook, stirring frequently, until the onions are softened. Sauté for 1 minute more after adding the garlic.

2. Stir in the tomatoes, chicken strips, and curry powder. Cook, stirring constantly, for about 10-15 minutes, or until the chicken is thoroughly cooked and the mixture is thick.

3. Stir in the coconut milk and cook for another 5 minutes.

4. Sprinkle with cinnamon and garnish with basil. Serve immediately with plain rice or nutty green rice.

CRISPY RICE SQUARES

Makes 32 squares

1 teaspoon coconut oil, cold-pressed

½ cup brown rice syrup

2 tbsp. almond butter

1 tsp vanilla extract

2 cup crunchy brown rice cereal

2 cups puffed rice

2 cups puffed millet

½ cup pumpkin or sunflower seeds

½ cup currants, dried apples, or dates

Directions

1. In a large pot, heat the oil. Mix in the rice syrup and almond butter. Stir until it is bubbly.

2. Remove from the heat and stir in the vanilla extract.

3. Stir in the remaining ingredients with a wooden spoon.

4. Press mixture flat in an ungreased 9"x13" pan. Allow the mixture to cool at room temperature or refrigerate.

5. Cut the dough into squares. Keep it in an airtight container.

Tips: Substitutions include agave syrup or honey in place of brown rice syrup, tahini in place of almond butter, currents or dates in place of dried apples, and grape seed oil in place of coconut oil.

EVERYDAY BASIC VINAIGRETTE

8 servings

¼ cup vinegar of choice

3 tablespoons lemon juice

1 clove garlic (or 1 teaspoon minced garlic)

½ teaspoon cumin

1 tbsp raw honey

1 teaspoon Dijon mustard

½ teaspoon sea salt

¼ teaspoon pepper

1-2 tablespoons fresh minced parsley

2-4 chopped green onions

¼ cup extra-virgin olive oil

Directions

1. Blend the vinegar, lemon juice, garlic, cumin, honey, mustard, sea salt, and pepper in a blender.

2. Stir in the fresh chopped parsley and onion.

3. Blend in the oil (if possible, slowly stream in oil through an opening in the top of the blender).

4. Serve at room temperature.

For a different flavor blend, replace the cumin with 12 to 1 teaspoon dried basil or 1-2 tablespoons fresh basil.

FRESH BERRIES WITH COCONUT MANGO CREAM

4 servings

⅔ cup canned coconut milk (canned)

1⅓ cup frozen diced mango (do not defrost)

1 teaspoon vanilla extract

2 cup blueberries or blackberries, fresh

4 mint leaves to garnish (optional)

Directions

1. Place the coconut milk and frozen mango in a blender. On high, blend until smooth.

2. Blend in the vanilla extract for a few seconds more.

3. Divide the berries evenly among four dishes. Serve topped with coconut cream.

4. Optionally garnish with a mint leaf.

Add ⅓ cup frozen raspberries to the coconut milk and mango for a variation. The pink color contrasts beautifully with the berries.

FRUITY SPINACH SALAD

4 servings

1 pint organic fresh strawberries (or 2 cups sliced)

8 washed, dried, and ripped fresh spinach

Dressing:

1 tablespoon toasted sesame seeds

½ tablespoon poppy seeds

1 chopped scallion

1 tablespoon flax seed oil

1 tablespoon extra virgin olive oil

two tbsp balsamic vinegar

1 tablespoon sesame seeds for garnish

Directions

1. Cut the berries in half and arrange them in a serving bowl over the spinach.

2. In a blender or food processor, combine all of the dressing ingredients and process until smooth. Pour over salad and toss just before serving.

3. Garnish with nuts if desired.

Tips: For a different flavor, substitute raspberries for the strawberries and sliced almonds for the walnuts.

GUACAMOLE

4 servings

2 minced garlic cloves (2 teaspoons)

¼ cup minced scallions or red onion

¼ jalapeos, minced

2 peeled avocados

1 tablespoon fresh lime juice (12 lime juice)

2 tablespoon fresh cilantro, chopped

1 pinch of sea salt

Directions

1. Combine the garlic, scallions, and jalapeos in a medium mixing bowl.

2. Mash the avocado with the back of a fork.

3. Gently fold in the lime juice.

4. Garnish with cilantro and sea salt to taste.

KALE PINEAPPLE BANANA SMOOTHIE

2 servings

1½ cup almond or coconut milk, unsweetened

1 cup packed chopped kale

½ cup pineapple, diced or chunked, fresh, frozen, or canned in juice and drained

½ banana (frozen is best)

½ cup ice, optional

2 scoops vanilla vegan protein powder

1 tablespoon chia or ground flax seed

Rice, pea, and hemp are examples of common varieties. Should be sweetened with stevia or left unsweetened. 1 scoop should contain 17g of protein.

Directions

Blend all of the ingredients in a blender until smooth.

NUTTY GREEN RICE

8 servings

1 cup brown or basmati rice

14 tsp salt

2 cup water

½ cup sliced almonds

1 bunch fresh parsley

1 tsp garlic

1½ teaspoon lemon juice

1½ teaspoon olive oil

¼ tsp freshly ground pepper

½ diced cucumber for garnish

Directions

1. Bring the water to a boil, then add the rice and salt, stir, and cover for 45 minutes. Do not stir any further. Remove from heat and set aside for 10 minutes before removing the cover and allowing to cool.

2. In a food processor, combine almonds, parsley, garlic, pepper, and oil while the rice is cooking.

3. When the rice has cooled, combine it with the nut mixture.

4. If desired, garnish with cucumber.

OVEN–BAKED LENTIL AND SPLIT PEA SOUP

8 servings

1 cup well-rinsed split peas

1 cup well-rinsed lentils

10 cup vegetable broth (low sodium)

2 medium sliced or diced carrots

2 sliced or diced celery stalks

1 large chopped red bell pepper (1½-2 cup)

1 large chopped onion

1 bay leaf

¼ teaspoon ground black pepper 1 teaspoon cumin

½ teaspoon of salt

Directions

1.In a Dutch oven or large oven-proof pot, combine peas and lentils.

2.Add the remaining ingredients and bake, covered, for about 2 hours, or until the lentils and peas are tender.

3. Alternatively, cook on top of the stove for 1 hour, stirring occasionally. Before serving, remove the bay leaf.

OVEN-ROASTED VEGETABLES

4 servings

1 cup florets broccoli

1 cup florets cauliflower

1 carrot cup

1 cup sliced bell peppers

1 onion cup

1 cup of mushrooms

1 yellow squash cup

1 pound asparagus

¼ cup extra virgin olive oil

1 tbsp. minced garlic

½ teaspoon of salt

½ teaspoon black pepper, coarsely ground

Directions

1. While preparing the vegetables, preheat the oven to 375° F. Chop the vegetables so that they are all about the same size. This ensures that all vegetables finish cooking at the same time.

2. Toss all ingredients in a large roasting pan or cookie sheet and spread in a single layer.

3. Roast for 25-30 minutes, or until the vegetables are tender and slightly brown, stirring occasionally.

Tips: To make preparation easier, reduce the variety of vegetables but keep the total amount to 8 cups for nutritional consistency. You could, for example, chop 8 cups broccoli.

OVERNIGHT STEEL-CUT OATS

8 servings

6 cups water

½ teaspoon sea salt

1½ cup gluten-free steel cut oats

Directions

1. Bring water to a boil in a saucepan.

2. Mix in the salt and oats.

3. Cover and remove from heat. Place in the refrigerator on a hot pad and leave overnight.

4. In the morning, reheat the oatmeal over low heat. (You may need to add a little water to achieve the desired consistency).

5. Store leftovers in the refrigerator.

Tips: If your meal plan allows it, add small amounts of nuts, seeds, fruits, and spices as desired to add nutritional balance.

PUMPKIN OATMEAL PANCAKES

4 servings

1 cup gluten-free rolled oats plus 2 tablespoons

¼ teaspoon ginger powder

¼ teaspoon cinnamon

¼ teaspoon nutmeg

¼ teaspoon ground cloves or allspice

½ teaspoon of salt

½ tsp baking soda

⅔ cup pureed pumpkin

⅓ cup applesauce, unsweetened

⅓ cup unsweetened coconut milk or almond milk

2 tablespoons melted coconut oil

1 teaspoon maple syrup

1 tsp vanilla extract

2 tbsp ground flax seed and ⅔ cup water as an egg replacer

Directions

1. Make the egg replacer by combining ground flax and water. Allow 5 minutes for the mixture to gel.

2. In a high-speed blender, pulse the oats until finely ground, about 60 seconds. Combine the spices, salt, and baking soda in a mixing bowl.

3. In a separate bowl, combine the pumpkin, applesauce, milk, melted coconut oil, maple syrup, vanilla extract, and egg replacer. Stir the wet ingredients into the dry ingredients until just combined. Avoid over-mixing.

4. Heat a nonstick skillet or cast iron skillet over medium heat (or an electric griddle over 350° F). Oil or butter the surface lightly.

5. When the pan is hot, pour ¼ cup of the batter into it and gently spread the circles. Cook the pancake until bubbles form around the edges. These pancakes cook a little slower than regular pancakes, so keep the heat on

medium and give them some time. Cook for an additional 2 minutes on the other side.

2.Drizzle with organic agave nectar or maple syrup and serve warm. (Note, neither agave nor maple syrup were included in the nutrition analysis chart).

QUICK BROWN RICE AND BLACK BEAN BOWL

4 servings

4 teaspoon coconut oil

2 cup baby spinach, chopped

2 cups brown rice

2 cans rinsed and drained black beans

1 tablespoon of sea salt

1 garlic powder teaspoon

1 teaspoon cumin

1 chopped avocado

1 cup tomatoes, chopped

Directions

1. Melt the butter in a large skillet over medium-high heat. Melt the coconut oil in a saucepan. Sauté the spinach until wilted.

2. Combine the rice, beans, sea salt, garlic powder, and cumin in a mixing bowl. Cook until all of the ingredients are hot. Take off the heat.

3. Gently fold in the avocado and tomatoes just before serving.

QUINOA SALAD WITH CHICKEN, GRAPES, AND ALMONDS

8 servings

2 cups water

1¼ cup quinoa, red or brown

1 teaspoon vinegar (rice or balsamic)

1 tablespoon lemon juice

1 tbsp lime juice

¼ teaspoon sea salt

¼ teaspoon pepper

2 tbsp olive oil

½ cup fresh mint, chopped

½ cup fresh basil, chopped

¼ cup fresh cilantro, chopped

2 cups shredded chicken breast

2 cups grapes, halved

½ cup sliced and toasted almonds

3-4 cups baby spinach, chopped

½ cup chopped green onions

Directions

1. Rinse the quinoa under cold running water and drain. Bring 2 cups water to a boil, then add the quinoa and a pinch of salt. Reduce heat to low and simmer for 12-15 minutes, or until most of the liquid has been absorbed. Uncover and set aside to cool.

2. In a large mixing bowl, combine vinegar, lemon and lime juices, sea salt, and pepper. Slowly drizzle in the olive oil and freshly chopped herbs. Mix thoroughly.

3. Toss cooled quinoa with dressing. Toss in the chicken, grapes, nuts, baby spinach, and green onions.

4. Serve at room temperature or chilled, if desired.

Tips: If desired, have the chicken cooked and shredded or chopped ahead of time. For presentation, serve on a lettuce leaf. For a colorful presentation, combine red quinoa and green grapes or regular quinoa and red grapes.

ROASTED PECANS AND FRESH PEARS WITH MIXED GREENS

4 servings

½ cup raw pecans

4 cups mixed greens of choice (spring mix, baby spinach, or arugula)

¼ red onion, thinly sliced in rounds, cut in half

1 ripe pear

Vinaigrette:

2 tablespoons vinegar of choice

½ lemon juice (1.5 tbsp)

½ clove garlic (or 12 teaspoon minced garlic)

14 teaspoon cumin

½ tbsp raw honey

½ teaspoon Dijon mustard

¼ teaspoon sea salt

⅛ teaspoon pepper

1 tablespoon fresh minced parsley

2 chopped green onions

2 tbsp extra-virgin olive oil

Directions

1. Roast raw pecans in a 350°F oven for 5-8 minutes, or until browned. Be careful not to burn the nuts.

2. Toss greens and onions together in a large salad bowl.

3. Garnish with cooled roasted pecans.

4. Just before serving, peel pears, cut into chunks, and place on top of salad.

5. Toss all of the other ingredients right before serving, and top with either variation of the Everyday Basic Vinaigrette below.

Everyday Basic Vinaigrette:

1 Combine the vinegar, lemon juice, garlic, cumin, honey, mustard, sea salt, and pepper in a blender and blend.

2. Stir in the fresh chopped parsley and onion.

3. Blend in the oil (if possible, slowly stream in oil through an opening in the top of the blender).

4. Serve at room temperature.

For a different flavor blend, replace the cumin with ½ to 1 teaspoon dried basil or 1-2 tablespoons fresh basil.

SAGE TURKEY SAUSAGE

4 servings (This recipe makes 8 patties.)

1 pound turkey breast ground

¼ cup apple, finely diced

2 tbsp red onion, finely minced

2 tbsp fresh sage, finely minced

½ teaspoon fresh thyme, finely minced

3 tbsp extra-virgin olive oil

½ tsp kosher salt

½ teaspoon black pepper, freshly ground

Directions

1. Combine turkey, apple, onion, sage, thyme, 1 tablespoon olive oil, salt, and pepper in a large mixing bowl.

2. Form the turkey mixture into eight patties.

3. Melt butter in a nonstick skillet over medium heat. Mix in 2 tablespoons olive oil.

4. Brown the patties on each side for 3-4 minutes, or until firm to the touch.

5. Refrigerate leftovers in an airtight glass container for up to 3 days.

SAUTÉED SESAME GREEN BEANS

4 servings

1 pound fresh or frozen petite green beans

1 tbsp olive oil (extra virgin)

2 garlic cloves (or 2 teaspoons minced garlic)

1 tablespoon basil, fresh (or 1 teaspoon dried)

1 tablespoon sesame seeds, roasted

1 teaspoon coarse sea salt

½ teaspoon black pepper, or to taste

Directions

1. Steam green beans for 7-8 minutes in a steamer basket over water. Remove from heat and drain when they are bright green and fork tender. Place aside.

2. Preheat a large skillet over medium heat. Sauté the olive oil and garlic for about 2-3 minutes. Garlic should be slightly browned, but not burned.

3. Add steamed green beans to pan and cook until warm and coated with olive oil and garlic.

4. Turn off the heat. Toss with basil, roasted sesame seeds, salt, and pepper right away. Serve hot.

Tips: This dish is delicious as leftovers.

SAVORY SEED CRACKERS

8 servings

⅓ cup chia seeds

⅓ cup flax seeds

⅓ cup sunflower seeds

¼ cup water

⅛ teaspoon garlic powder

⅛ teaspoon onion powder

¼ teaspoon salt

¼ teaspoon guar or xanthan gum

If needed, add more water.

Directions

1. Preheat the oven to 300° F.

2. Combine all of the ingredients and spread on a cookie sheet lined with greased parchment paper. Press flat (about ⅛-inch thick).

3. Bake for 30 minutes on each side.

4. Score the seeds immediately after removing them from the oven (they will still be pliable at this point, but score right away, as they will firm up quickly). A pizza cutter works well.

To prevent seeds from sticking to your hands, oil your hands or a spatula before spreading on a cookie sheet. Take care not to burn the seeds. Consider cooking for a longer period of time at a lower cooking temperature (i.e., 250° F).

SIMPLE ROASTED BUTTERNUT SQUASH

4 servings

4 cups butternut squash cubes

2 tbsp of olive oil

2 minced garlic cloves

¼ teaspoon salt

¼ teaspoon pepper

Directions

1. Preheat the oven to 400°F

2. Toss butternut squash, olive oil, garlic, salt, and pepper in a large mixing bowl.

3. Arrange coated squash in a single layer on a baking sheet.

4. Roast the squash at 400°F until tender and lightly browned (about 25-30 minutes).

STRAWBERRY MANGO SMOOTHIE

2 servings

2 cups unsweetened almond, hemp, or coconut milk

1 cup frozen strawberries (no sugar added)

1 cup frozen mangoes (no sugar added)

2 scoops vanilla vegan protein powder*

2 tablespoons chia seeds

2 cups spinach leaves

Soy-free. Rice, peas, and hemp are examples of common varieties. Should be sweetened with stevia or left unsweetened entirely. 1 scoop should contain 17g protein.

Directions

1. Place all of the ingredients in a blender and blend until smooth.

SWEET POTATO AND KALE SOUP

4 servings

1 medium chopped onion

1 garlic clove minced

1 chopped red or yellow bell pepper

3 peeled and cubed medium sweet potatoes or yams

¼ teaspoon sea salt

¼ teaspoon freshly ground black pepper

5 cup low-sodium chicken or vegetable broth

1 liter coconut milk

1 bunch dinosaur kale, thinly sliced (about 5-6 cups)

Directions

1. Place the onion, garlic, bell peppers, sweet potatoes, and broth in a large soup pot. Bring everything to a boil. Reduce to a low heat and continue to cook for 5 minutes.

2. Cook for 3-4 minutes after adding coconut milk and kale.

3. The soup is done when all of the vegetables are soft.

Serve the soup with brown rice or quinoa as a side dish. For a low-carb meal, serve over cauliflower rice.

SWEET POTATO HUMMUS

8 servings

1 large sweet potato (12-14 ounces), cooked and mashed

1 can (15 ounces) rinsed and drained chick peas

¼ cup tahini

¼ cup lemon juice

3 tbsp extra virgin olive oil

1 small garlic clove, halved

1½ teaspoons coarse sea salt

1 teaspoon cumin powder

½ teaspoon ground cinnamon (optional)

Directions

1. Combine all of the ingredients in a blender or food processor. Blend until smooth.

Serve with vegetables or seed crackers as a side dish. To reduce sodium content per serving, cut the added sea salt in half, add some pepper, or increase the other spices to taste.

THREE BEAN VEGETABLE CHILI

6 servings

1 tbsp olive oil

12 large onion, diced

2 carrots, diced

1 red bell pepper, chopped

1 seeded and minced jalapeo pepper

1½ tbsp chili powder

2 teaspoon cumin powder

1½ teaspoon oregano

1 (28 ounce) can no-salt tomatoes, diced

1 quart water

1 (15 ounce) can rinsed and drained black beans

1 can (15 ounce) rinsed and drained red kidney beans

1 can (15 ounce) rinsed and drained Great Northern beans

½ teaspoon sea salt

Fresh cilantro as garnish

Scallions, finely chopped

Directions

1. Heat the oil in a large saucepan or stockpot over medium heat. Cook until onions, carrots, bell peppers, garlic, and jalapeo are translucent (about 5 minutes).

2. Cook for 1 minute, stirring frequently, with dry spices (chili powder, cumin, and oregano).

3. Pour in the canned tomatoes with juices, water, beans, and salt. Bring to a boil, then reduce to a low heat and leave to simmer for 30 minutes, uncovered.

4. Garnish with cilantro and scallions before serving.

Tips: Look for canned beans that are low in sodium. Otherwise, to reduce sodium, rinse beans thoroughly after draining.

WALNUT-CRUSTED FISH

4 servings

4 flounder fillets (4 ounces each)

¼ cup almond milk

1 cup walnuts, finely chopped

¼ teaspoon salt

¼ teaspoon black pepper

1½ tbsp extra virgin olive oil

1 tablespoon fresh lemon juice (1½ lemon juice)

¼ cup fresh chopped parsley for garnish

Directions

1. Rinse and pat dry the fish with a paper towel after rinsing it in cold water.

2. Fill a shallow bowl halfway with almond milk.

3. Arrange the walnuts, salt, and pepper on a plate.

4. Dredge the fish in the walnut mixture after dipping it in the almond milk. Gently press the walnuts onto the fish to form the crust.

5. Melt butter in a large skillet over medium heat. Then add the fish and olive oil. Cook for 3-4 minutes on each side, or until the fish is done.

6. Squeeze lemon juice over the top and top with parsley. Sole can also be used in place of flounder.

YELLOW RICE

8 servings

2 cups low-sodium chicken broth

1 small onion, finely chopped

2 teaspoon olive oil

1 garlic clove, minced

1 teaspoon turmeric

1 cup long-grain brown rice (uncooked)

Directions

1. In a 2-quart saucepan over low heat, sauté onions in oil until tender, about 5 minutes.

2. Cook for 1 minute after adding the garlic.

3. Stir in the turmeric, followed by the rice. Pour in the stock. Bring to a boil, then reduce to a low heat for 45 minutes, or until the rice is tender and the liquid has been absorbed. Do not stir.